Disclaimer

INTRODUCTION

With health knowledge and discoveries, it has been poised that health is wealth and one of the easiest ways to build and maintain good health is dieting. It's a key that can lengthen lives and build a good and healthy body structure and cells. dieting is the method of consuming a diet with an accountable attitude. Therefore, Dieting itself consists of varieties that make it more active and relevant to build a good and healthy body. Dieting is not just a dream it can be a reality and to make it a reality, a positive mindset for dieting should be fostered. While dieting, it's relevant to do it with the right reasons to achieve positive goals. It's not just an activity for adults but also forbidden. It's also a note to recognize that great mistakes are done by many while dieting, this is because of adopting an all-nothing attitude. Dieting is a great help and an aid to weight watchers. Lastly, it's necessary to acknowledge the fact that to engage in dieting, there are health tips that can help such as Drinking water in large quantities, setting up goals, and eating more.

Chapter 1

AN OVERVIEW OF DIETING AND HEALTH

Foxcroft claims that the word "diet" is derived from the Greek word "digital," which refers to a holistic idea of a balanced lifestyle that encompasses both mental and physical health rather than a specific weight-loss plan.

To lessen, conserve, or increase body weight, or to deter and deal with diseases like diabetes and obesity, dieting is the method of consuming a diet with an accountable attitude. People with weight-related health issues are advised to diet, but not everyone else.

The body's compartments design internally bottled energy references, like complicated carbs and lipids, for power when the body is utilizing extra energy than it is expanding (very as when exercising). Weight reduction is evident as a result of this process, which breaks down fat cells or adipose tissue.

It has been established that different calorie-reduced diets, such as those stressing particular macronutrients (low-fat, low-carbohydrate, etc.), are not more effective than one another because weight loss depends on calorie intake.

Long-term responsibility for food is the biggest pointer to achievement because strength regain is widespread. The findings of a diet might, nonetheless, differ vastly banking on the person.

The first well-liked eating plan was called "Banting," after William

Banting. He described the specific low-carb, low-calorie diet that had caused his significant weight loss in his 1863 pamphlet Letter on Corpulence, Addressed to the Public.

VARIETIES OF DIETING

Any diet can be categorized into one of these six groups based on its goal or mode of operation.

Low-fat

Reduced dietary fat content is a key component of low-fat diets. Less fat is consumed, which lowers calorie intake. It has been discovered that a low-fat, plant-based diet enhances blood sugar control, cardiovascular health, and weight management.

Low-carbohydrate

Diets short in carbohydrates incline to be elevated in protein and oil. "Diets founded on this analysis are named Low GI diets, and the most notable difference of this diet is the 'Paleo-diet,' which rates feeds established on their all-around effect on blood sugar levels.

Low-calorie

One of the vastly outstanding low-calorie diets is "Weight Watchers," which frequently concludes in an energy shortage of 500-1,000 calories per day, which can steer to a 0.5 to 1 kilogram (1.1 to 2.2 pounds) weight loss each week.

ultra-low calorie

Very low-calorie diets subject the body to starvation and result in an average loss of 1.5-2.5 kg (3.3-5.5 lb) per week. "2-4-6-8", a prominent diet of this species, attends a four-day cycle in which only 200 calories are expended on the first day, 400 on the second day, 600 on the third day, 800 on the fourth day, and again completely fasting.

Fasting

Long-term (periodic) fasting is not advised in dieting; instead, eating little and often is encouraged. Long-term fasting is risky since it increases the risk of malnutrition and should only be done under medical supervision. Intermittent fasting is the most common type of this diet.

Detox

Many of these diets include herbs or celery and other juicy low-calorie veggies and are pushed with unfounded claims that they may remove "toxins" from the human body.

Dietary Success Factors:

Taking care of these issues will enable you to achieve the best results and maintain your diet for a longer period, regardless of the technique of dieting you select.

Recent research suggests that innovative scheduling techniques, such as intermittent fasting or missing meals, and carefully placing snacks before meals, may be advised.

Food Journaling: A 2008 study found that dieters who kept a daily food journal (or diet notebook) lost twice as much weight as those who did not. This finding raises the possibility that people who keep a food journal are more mindful of what they eat and hence consume fewer calories.

Water: A 2009 analysis found scant evidence that boosting water drinking and switching to calorie-free drinks instead of alcoholic ones (i.e., consuming fewer calories) may help with weight management.

Chapter 2

DIETING FOR HEALTH

Nothing motivates you to diet more than your health and well-being. The hazards and potential outcomes that may emerge from our weight are something those of us who are overweight are more aware of than

others. However, until we reach our turning point, the hazards may not often appear as clear-cut as they are for smokers.
Until you entirely modify your eating habits and lifestyle choices, nothing will change, regardless of whether your eating patterns are the result of an addiction to particular foods, an emotional need, or years of taught behavior and conditioning.

For many individuals, dieting has taken on a life of its own. People often switch between diets, or yo-yo, with little success and increasing despondency at the utter lack of progress. The reality is that no diet will be effective unless you decide to forget about your mistakes and immediately get back on track. Simple dietary changes won't make the pounds instantly vanish, and denying yourself the foods you love may have more negative effects than favorable ones.

The most important lesson that the majority of people need to understand is that dieting isn't always beneficial.

The majority of overweight individuals require positive lifestyle adjustments most of all, thus they should prioritize implementing them into their daily routines. People laugh at the idea of using the stairs or finding a parking spot farther away, but they are also completely reasonable ways to get in a little extra physical exercise each day. If none of those work for you, how about taking up dancing? If you're ready to put in the effort, there are beginner dance classes in most areas that will accept and invite dancers of all ages, sizes, and fitness abilities. What a fantastic way to stay in shape, discover something new and enjoy yourself without going hungry.

Another fantastic benefit of an activity like dance class is that, in most situations, you are not eating or tempted to eat while you are dancing (imagine ballroom dancing with your significant other). You are burning the calories you did not consume, which is another fantastic thing. Try joining a walking group or picking up another pastime if dancing isn't your thing.

When it comes to dieting and weight reduction, anything that gets you up and moving and away from the temptation of your refrigerator is a good thing. Significant weight loss is not possible with diet alone. If you want to get the quick and impressive results that many dieters are looking for, you must add physical activity to your daily regimen.

Another problem with dieting is that many individuals give up too soon.

People give up midway through the process or become frustrated that they aren't losing enough weight dramatically as quickly as they had hoped, marking off yet another failure when they could have succeeded more than ever before if they had stuck with their original diet plan for a little while longer.

Another thing to keep in mind while dieting is that the scale may either be your greatest friend or your worst adversary. You are setting yourself up for failure if you weigh yourself every day in the anticipation of seeing the scale drop another pound. If you are having depressed episodes of Rocky Road or Chunky Monkey every night because you didn't shed 10 pounds overnight, you will never get the results you want.

There aren't many diets that work when it comes to weight loss. There are, however, a lot of lifestyle adjustments that, when applied regularly and assiduously, have positive results. It's important to keep in mind that you must put in the effort since it is quite improbable that any diet would.

Chapter 3

MAKING DIETING A REALITY

Dieting is far too often approached from the mindset of impending failure. Too many people have tried and failed so many diets in the past that they try the next new diet with the absolute knowledge that they will fail in this attempt as well. Guess what? They will.

Henry Ford once said, “If you think you can or think you can’t you will always be right.” If you think you are going to fail at this diet you are dooming yourself to failure before you even deprive yourself of the first bite. Think about that before you begin because only a true masochist could find pleasure in perpetuating this vicious cycle without ever stopping to wonder why none of the other diets have worked for you. Henry Ford also said, “Failure is only the opportunity to begin again more intelligently”. In case you were wondering I would say his words are quite profound. Seriously though, if you do not examine the reasons for your failures you are certainly dooming yourself to repeat them, and if you are already planning to fail why on earth would you even try?

You are the only person who can take control of your need to eat. You are the only one who can pay attention and notice when you are eating for emotional fulfillment and when you are eating from necessity. You and you alone can get yourself out of your chair and on your feet. You are the only one that can take the responsibility for the condition in which you find yourself. There are medical exceptions but even in these situations if you are trying diet after diet and failing over and over again then you must at some point in time realize that it is quite likely not the diets that aren't working.

We must all be accountable for our successes and failures in life. It is no different when it comes to dieting. There are few better feelings in the world than for someone to notice and compliment your efforts. If you are very obese, unfortunately, it may take a little more time for people to notice the weight you've lost. Too many men and women give up simply because no one noticed and that is an incredible shame. Allow your dieting practices to work before you decide they are a failure and you just might surprise yourself with a roaring success.

The truth is far too few people hold themselves accountable to their dieting and weight loss goals. This means that far too many people are giving up without really ever bothering to give it an effort. If you have an issue holding yourself accountable to your dieting plans, perhaps you would do well to diet with a partner. This helps you not only set goals but also meet and exceed challenges along the way. A partner can also benefit from the partnership as he or she will be challenged and feel the need to perform better than if he or she were dieting alone.

You must hold yourself accountable to your stated dieting and weight loss goals to achieve lasting results. If you have not had dieting success in the past, then perhaps it is time to bring some degree of accountability into the picture and make it happen.

Chapter 4

DIETING MINDSET

When it comes to dieting, far too many people set themselves up for failure before they even begin the process. They dread going on their diets and before they start the process are planning their mishaps along the way. Sad to say but true, far too many would-be dieters are planning their first Rocky Road mishap while eating their last bowl of Rocky Road before the big event.

I have no idea why we tend to do this to ourselves but it is something I see in dieters everywhere. The far too popular notion is that one must binge on the foods most loved and enjoyed before beginning the dieting process because these things must be eliminated to shed those unwanted pounds. If you are honest with yourself, nothing could be further from the truth. Moderation is simply a concept that many of us are loathe to embrace.

You must change your way of thinking about food and your enjoyment of food for any diet you embrace to be successful. Food isn't the enemy. And that is something that not enough people understand. Even the 'tasty' foods aren't the enemy. The enemy is your inability to properly portion the foods you eat.

The problem is that the vast majority of us eat the wrong foods far more often than we eat the right foods. This is where the problems lie.

Our bodies need the nutrients we are lacking by not eating the five servings of vegetables and three servings of fruit each day that we should consume. Our bodies know that something is missing and we feel hungry or deprived. If we were consuming the proper balance of fruits and veggies each day we would find that we were far less likely to feel hungry and desire those foods that aren't as healthy. This means we would be much more likely to enjoy them in moderation as they should be enjoyed.

Portion control is another problem that we have. We live in a society of “upselling”. Super-sized fries and empty calories by the gallon of your favorite cola are offered with almost every fast food meal that can be bought.

You must learn to say no to these things and avoid situations in which you may feel tempted to partake in these upsized orders.

To be truly successful when dieting you need to embrace the process of building a healthier you rather than depriving yourself of something. Do not think of your weight loss plan as something negative but rather as a positive force in your life to make changes for the better. When you have negative thoughts do not direct them to your diet. When you feel deprived, remind yourself that you are depriving your bones of carrying around that excess weight. Remind yourself that you are depriving your wardrobe of those bulky clothes that are designed to hide the bulges.

Remind yourself that you are depriving your body of years of bulges and bringing back the body of your youth.

Do not get so caught up in the dieting process that you forget to enjoy some of the goodies that life has to offer. Watching your weight and counting your calories does not mean that you can never go over your allotment. The goal however is to find balance. If you learn to portion your food correctly, indulge in moderation, and incorporate enjoyable calorie-burning activities into your daily routine you may be amazed at the results.

Dieting for weight loss and health is only depriving if you allow it to be. If you cannot control yourself when it comes to indulging then by all means avoid indulging. However, if you can learn to incorporate those small treats into your routine in moderation and burn those extra calories as well, then you should find yourself a much happier and more successful 'dieter' than you have ever managed to be in the past.

Chapter 5

DIETING FOR THE RIGHT REASONS

When it comes to dieting, far too often we take those first steps towards weight loss bliss for what we later determine are all the wrong reasons. Ultimately, however, if your reason works for you there is no truly wrong reason to diet. The trick is in finding the reason that will work for you.

I've seen all kinds of excellent motivators when it comes to dieting and taking your diet seriously. One of the more common reasons is to lose weight. This is as good of a reason as any. Some want to get back into the size 5 jeans they wore in high school while others would simply like to be able to look in the mirror once again without feeling guilty. For some, this is a simple matter of vanity and for others, it is finally managing to deal with what has become a lifelong problem. If you find the inspiration you need to be successful with your dieting this time as opposed to others, then that is the perfectly plausible and acceptable reason for you to diet.

Other reasons for dieting include a desire to be more physically fit. Some of us have a deep and abiding desire to live as long as possible and firmly believe that the best possible method for accomplishing this goal is to live the healthiest life possible. This is another excellent reason for losing weight and getting into shape. If it works for you that is. The thing to remember is that every person is going to have to find their very own motivation deep within.

Yet another great reason is to have the energy you need to keep up with your little ones. This is one of the heartbreaking side effects for most when it comes to obesity. There is simply no energy left over at the end of the day to enjoy doing things with your precious little ones who are young for such a very short amount of time. You desperately want to be able to build those precious memories with them but have no energy with which to do so. If that isn't bad enough you probably (if you are considered morbidly obese) have noticed that many of the simplest activities with your children often bring you physical pain that is the direct result of your weight.

Revenge is a dish that is best served cold and another excellent motivator for some when it comes to dieting and taking off those pesky pounds. Losing a great deal of weight takes time in many cases so you must be able to maintain your motivation even when things are going rough along the way. The path to a new body is not easy. This is for those who have some serious emotional healing to do and the best revenge for old slights and wounds is to come back more beautiful than ever before. If this motivation is what it takes for you to take off the pounds then this is the motivation to which you should cling.

Religion is another common weight loss motivation. Some people believe the body should be treated as a temple. There is nothing wrong with this philosophy at all, though it takes some of us longer to find our way to that line of thinking than others. Religion and faith are powerful motivators, as they have been known to bring healing to those in need through the power of their faith or their prayers. If your faith can give you the willpower and strength you need to reach your dieting and weight loss goals then by all means lean on your faith and hold it close.

No matter what motivation you have for dieting and losing weight if you find it is no longer working for you, then you need to find another motivator quickly. Without proper motivation, it is quite unlikely that you will ever meet your weight loss goals.

Chapter 6

SETTING GOALS WHEN DIETING

As with most things in life, setting goals is very important when dieting. When you look at things truthfully and objectively you should notice that most of the things you've accomplished in life have been accomplished because you not only had a goal but also had a planned and well-thought-out process for achieving that goal. That being said, why is goal setting so important when it comes to dieting?

First of all, it is difficult to achieve a goal if you do not have a clearly defined goal. There are times in life when it is almost impossible to tell whether you are succeeding or failing because you aren't certain exactly what the desired outcome should be. Identifying your dieting goals before you begin eliminates this particular possibility.

Second, having dieting goals gives you a measuring stick by which you can judge your process. This is important so that you know when your efforts are falling behind and when you're moving along schedule or ahead of schedule. In other words, you will know when to celebrate and when to give yourself a swift kick to the rear.

Now that we know why we set weight loss goals, let's discuss how we should go about setting those goals that are so important for dieting success. You want to set aggressive goals without being impossible to achieve. If you set goals that are beyond your reach you will find that frustration will be your dieting partner until you reach the point where you give up together. To avoid this you should take great care to ensure that your goals are possible for you to achieve.

When it comes to weight loss be specific when setting your goals. Rather than setting a total goal of 40 or 60 pounds start with a specific goal such as 10 pounds in one month. Then you can extend the goal to the next month until you've reached the overall goal of 40 or 60 pounds. It is much easier to lose 10 pounds four times than it is to lose 40 pounds at once. It's a trick of the mind but it works. Ten pounds sounds simple and achievable. Forty pounds sounds like an insurmountable obstacle.

Another thing about goals is that you want to hold yourself accountable but you shouldn't call the whole thing off if you only lose 9 pounds instead of 10. Instead, find out where you dropped the ball for the final pound and set your 10-pound goal for the next month.

You should also take great care that you are working with your personal goals and not the goals that someone else is pushing on you. The truth is that if it’s personal to you, it will be much more rewarding than if you are doing this for someone else. If your heart isn’t in it, there are very few goals that are going to motivate you properly.

Finally, you should establish small (non-food) rewards for accomplishing your dieting goals. Perhaps your reward will be a new accessory for your new (or new old) wardrobe or a pedicure for your new look. Make your reward something fun and frivolous and teach yourself that accomplishing your goals can be accomplished by something other than food. This is a key to dieting successfully.

Chapter 7

DIETING AND DIABETES

Very few people realize the profound effect that weight has on diabetes. Even instances of gestational diabetes are much greater in patients that are overweight than in those that are not. Type 2, or adult-onset diabetes is more commonly found in overweight people than those that are within their 'ideal' weight ranges. Almost 90% of those with Type 2 diabetes are overweight. If you are suffering from Type 2 diabetes, the best gift you could give yourself just might be the gift of getting your weight under control.

Among those that suffer from Type 2 diabetes almost 40% have high blood pressure, which is another condition that is believed to be exacerbated by excess weight. Being overweight might also lead to a condition known as insulin resistance in which the body no longer responds to the insulin that is needed to assist the body in using sugar and glucose as fuel on a cellular level.

There are some things you can do to help yourself out if you have been diagnosed with Type 2 diabetes or labeled at risk for this devastating condition.

First of all, take off the pounds.

I know this is much easier said than done. Dieting is never easy and rarely fun for the average person. However, if you do not begin to take drastic steps toward procuring the best possible health for yourself you may not be able to enjoy the quality of life you had planned for your golden years.

Let your condition be your motivation and make plans to enjoy watching your grandchildren and great-grandchildren graduate college.

Fight it standing up.

Don't sit down and let Diabetes control you. Stand up and take control of your body back. This is a fight to the finish and if you let it, diabetes will be your end. If you fight it stand up, lose weight, get out there and exercise, listen to the doctor's orders and follow them. Find the strength within you to battle this disease head-on. You'll be amazed at what happens when you decide to stand up and fight for your health.

Get active.

Find activities that you enjoy and get out there and do them. Don't make those activities passive activities either. Even if it's just going out to play shuffleboard every day, get out there and play. Enjoy your time in the sun. Pick flowers with the little ones. Take up golf. Do whatever it takes to get up and move every day to remember why you want to live forever in the first place.

Watch what you eat.

Garbage in, garbage out, right? You have strict dietary requirements once you've been diagnosed with diabetes. This means that you absolutely must follow your dietary restrictions. Learn to live within those limits to live and enjoy life to the fullest you can. The amazing thing is that there are all kinds of foods available that are friendly to those with diabetes that weren't around just a few short years ago. It is quite possible to live and eat quite nicely with diabetes if you stick to your plan. The most important thing about dieting with diabetes is that you never lose sight of how crucial it is to do so.

Chapter 8

DIETING FOR CHILDREN

It is difficult in the world we live in to watch as so many children overburden their bodies at such young ages by being overweight. These children simply cannot run, jump, and play with the other children because their bodies simply will not allow them to do so. For these children, dieting is almost a necessity despite our best efforts to insulate them from the self-esteem issues that often accompany obesity.

If you have a child that is well outside the normal weight range for his or her age you are the one who must make the efforts and take the necessary steps to insure they shed those pounds to live a life that is as close to normal as possible. The first thing you need to do however is consulted with your child's doctor about the best possible course of action that will also safeguard the health of your child.

Put quite frankly, however, if you do not take the effort to assist your child in shedding those pounds you are placing the health of your child at risk. We do not let our children play in the street, we don't let them run with knives, why on earth would we allow them to commit suicide with Twinkies? If you have a child that is overweight, the following tips should help you and them with their dieting.

First of all, do not make food a punishment or a reward. Food is part of the problem with your children and you do not need to use it against them. Instead, introduce them to healthy alternatives. Do not keep the junk in the house and do not let them purchase lunch at school. Pack their lunches for school so that you know what they are eating. If you don't give them junk food they cannot have it when at home and you can work to ensure that they can't get their hands on junk food when they leave the house.

Incorporate healthy snacks into your family's eating plan rather than junk food. Fresh fruit, cut-up vegetables, nuts, and frozen yogurt are good healthy snacks for your kids. When in doubt consult the food pyramid but watch calories in the process. You want your children to eat a well-balanced diet while eliminating junk food and sweets for the best result.

Cut out the juices and pop. This may be a huge ordeal in your house but the greatest gift you can offer your child is a deep and abiding appreciation for water. Water works to make their bellies feel full and keeps them hydrated for the added activities you should be introducing into their routines.

Have them take dance, take up a sport, or simply get out and run around the yard. The worst thing you can do is to allow your children to become comatose television, computer, or video game zombies. Get them out and get them active. This helps in two ways. First of all, they aren't eating if they are outside playing and having a good time. Second, they are burning calories as they play which is a huge bonus in the dieting process for your children.

As your child begins to take off the weight you should begin to notice a very profound difference in not only the way he or she carries himself or herself but also in his or her interactions with others. Your child will experience restored and renewed self-confidence as the pounds come off and the teasing at school stops.

If you are at a complete loss as to how to help your child take the weight off there are camps that are designed specifically to deal with weight issues and building self-esteem in children ages 7-19. One of these camps may be just the answer you are looking for. Another thing to consider is to lead by example. If you don't eat junk food, if you are active, and if you do not engage in emotional overeating your child will not be learning those behaviors from you or having them reinforced by you.

Chapter 9

GREAT DIETING MISTAKES

When it comes to dieting many mistakes are made on a near-daily basis. While many real profound mistakes go along with the territory there are a few that seem to have far more profound and lasting implications than others. Hopefully, by learning about these mistakes you can learn to avoid them in your weight-loss pursuits.

Perhaps the single largest mistake that dieters make is adopting an all-or-nothing attitude. These are the dieters that scour the pantry and the refrigerator removing anything that could be seen as a potential source of temptation. They embark on a dietary regimen that is nearly impossible to maintain and believe that all is lost the moment they stray from the strict guidelines of their diet.

While this may work for some in the short term, it sets them up for failure, frustration, and ill will towards the entire dieting process. The important thing when it comes to dieting is the goal. Your goal is to shed pounds.

There are many ways in which this can be done that do not require starving yourself or punishing yourself in the process.

Another great mistake when it comes to dieting is selecting a diet plan where you eat the same thing every day. Despite our human need for structure and routine we tend to enjoy changing our lunch routine on occasion. Select a diet or new nutrition plan that allows you to enjoy a wide variety of foods rather than one that limits you to the same meal or meal selection day in and day out.

Other common mistakes include depriving yourself of everything you enjoy. One thing that we often forget is the importance of moderation. Fill up on servings of fruits and vegetables but allow yourself to enjoy the occasional indulgence for the sake of sanity. If you never allow yourself to enjoy a taste of chocolate, why on earth would you want to live forever? Seriously, do not forget to enjoy food for the sake of dieting. There is nothing wrong or sinful about enjoying food. The problem lies when you enjoy only the wrong sorts of foods.

You should also avoid the mistake of not setting goals. While you do not want to set goals that are impossible to achieve you should also avoid the opposite end of the spectrum, which involves having no goals at all. Those who set aggressive and achievable goals will see the greatest degree of success. Making those goals public and asking for support is another thing that will help you achieve greater success. This is one reason the Weight Watchers program has enjoyed phenomenal success.

The final mistake when it comes to dieting that is made all too often is giving up. We all have setbacks along the way. Even those who have achieved monumental dieting success have met with failure on the road. The result, however, for those who stick with the plan is a healthier body and that is worth fighting for. Your goals may get sidetracked but you can set new goals. You may have had a bad day or even a bad week when it comes to your dietary goals and plans. Do not let this defeat your desire to become a healthier you.

Learn to overcome those mistakes and move on from them. Let your failures teach you as much as your successes and you should be well on your way to the healthier person that you know is hiding inside. Whether you want to get rid of 10 pounds or 210 pounds the only way to achieve that goal and make it last is by dedicating yourself to the process of becoming a healthier person.

A healthy person has healthy eating habits and doesn't starve him or herself. Nor does a healthy person binge on things that aren't healthy. Learn to enjoy food in moderation and you should be well on your way to the success you seek.

Chapter 10

WEIGHT WATCHERS DIETING

When it comes to dieting there are very few organizations that have achieved the lasting success of Weight Watchers. They have been around quite a while and show no signs of stopping. More importantly, their success stories speak volumes for those who join and stick with the program. So what makes this program so successful when many others come and go?

Community

Believe it or not, one of the most important things about Weight Watchers' secret to success, so to speak, is the sense of community that is forged between the men and women who are trying to lose weight. There is something humbling and exciting about standing in front of the scale week after week and sharing not only your successes and failures but also the failures and successes of others.

Far too often those who are dieting simply do not have an adequate support system at home. The bonding that is done during the Weight Watchers meeting is a strong bond of men and women who may come from different backgrounds and walks of life but who share a common goal for their futures-weight loss and better health. That is not a bond to be taken lightly particularly when they laugh and cry together. They are on their way going through the trenches together and the success of this type of program for motivating and encouraging is nothing short of phenomenal.

Evolution

Weight Watchers have a pattern for success but they are not beyond evolving with the needs of the time. While they will be the first to state that the most successful participants typically attend the meetings, Weight Watchers also offers alternatives for those with busy schedules and even those that are simply too afraid to go to the meetings. For these people there is the anonymity of online forums, message boards, and support groups.

Weight Watchers hasn't limited its evolutionary process to this alone, they've also in recent years added a points system that allows dieters participating in their program to more easily gauge how well they are doing by their dietary standards and requirements without needing to count every single calorie or weighing their food. We live in a world of busy people and it is often more hassle than many dieters find to be worth the effort to count every single calorie (particularly when dining out).

The Weight Watchers website is another example of their commitment to evolving and accommodating the diverse needs of the men and women participating in their program. If you haven't checked it out in a while you really should take a look and see what amazing insights and information they have to offer.

Commitment to Fitness

Weight Watchers know that it isn't just diet that gets results. When you combine diet with exercise the results are much more immediate and more profound. The fact that Weight Watchers stresses the importance of exercise and physical fitness in addition to proper nutrition and changing your way of thinking when it comes to food is yet another reason for their widely known success.

Weight Watchers is just one of much different weight loss and dieting programs in the market today. The fact that they have made a name for themselves and stand out above the rest in many ways is nothing to take lightly. It seems that there is a new weight loss program cropping up every other month or so and yet Weight Watchers continues to achieve visible and sustainable results in those who work the program. Very few programs can make that claim for as long as Weight Watchers has been able to.

When you combine all of the things mentioned above with the pre-packaged foods that are offered by Weight Watchers, the extensive recipes that are available for Weight Watcher's participants, and a solid track record for success you would be robbing yourself of the potential for lasting success if you didn't at least see what the plan has to offer you.

Chapter 11

DIETING FOR WEIGHT LOSS

Weight loss is the primary justification given today for dieting. The vast majority of us are dieting for vanity, even though the majority of us would love to claim the lofty banner of dieting for health. But this is a completely valid and believable justification for altering one's lifestyle to lose weight. This motivation may be stronger than many of the other frequently cited reasons for dieting.

One of the most common complaints among people on diets to lose weight is that they feel hungry all the time. You might wish to include some of the following tactics in your dieting regimen to assist in combat this. Eat more high-fiber foods to start. Numerous morning bowls of cereal, whole grains, apples, pears, and lima beans are excellent sources of fiber. However, fiber is often overused since, although it may be filling, it can also have some unfavorable side effects (remember that beans are a good source of fiber). When taking higher doses of fiber, consider utilizing a product like Beano. You may also experiment with ingesting more fiber throughout the day as opposed to all of it at once.

Drinking lots of water when dieting is another way to feel fuller while on a diet. When it comes to getting all the nutrients to their proper locations, water plays a critical role in the body. Additionally, water aids in the regulation of your metabolism, which is crucial to the process of dieting and weight loss. Additionally, drinking water will keep your skin supple so that if serious weight reduction starts, your skin will be easier to put back in place.

Gain portion control skills. We no longer understand what a proper portion looks like because servings are overinflated and supersized so frequently. Before salads, soups, appetizers, or desserts are purchased, restaurant meals are frequently more than enough for at least two complete meals. Your daily calorie intake can be tremendously overloaded if you don't learn how to portion food properly. Additionally, it can encourage you to consume larger portions of lower-calorie items like lettuce and other vegetables rather than calorie-dense carbohydrates or fried things.

Don't be a "Gung Ho." The capacity of the body and intellect has its limits. When you start a diet, your body's caloric intake is drastically altered. Overextending yourself can put your health at risk. Instead of approaching your diet with an all-or-nothing mentality, start by gradually reducing your caloric intake and making adjustments as you go. Going overboard with your diet plans increases the likelihood that your diet will fail.

For the best results, approach your diet step-by-step and add more physical exercise to the mix. Cleaning the house, playing with the kids, and even gardening may burn calories when done frequently. Instead of driving to the park or the corner store, walk there. While you're walking, pull a wagon or push a stroller. The increased weight will provide just enough resistance to cause an increase in calorie burning.

Although going on a diet to lose weight doesn't necessarily require you to make a big sacrifice, it will require a drastic shift in lifestyle if you want to shed more than a few extra pounds for vanity. No matter how thrilled you are with the new body hidden inside your old one, the health implications of losing weight are quite important and are well worth the effort.

Chapter 12
DIETING AND FITNESS

Two components must be present for one to live a long and healthy life: nutrition and exercise. Even while some people think they are all one thing, it couldn't be more than the truth. It is very feasible to have an excellent diet and poor exercise habits. It is also possible to have less-than-ideal eating habits while yet being quite physically active.

When Jimmy Buffet's "woman" is bemoaning something, she sings this smart little line:

"I revere my body as a sanctuary."

Yours is handled like a tent.

When I consider all the individuals who are following these "garbage in, garbage out" diets to lose weight as successfully as the ones who are promoting these goods, I can't help but think of this quote.

To be very honest, weight loss may be accomplished only by nutrition. It is challenging, but it is doable. It is also feasible to remain physically fit while carrying a few excess pounds. We are, in great part, what we consume. If we eat a diet that is heavy in fat and poor in other nutrients, our bodies won't have the energy they need to burn the fat. However, no matter how many weights we lift, if we aren't giving our body the resources it needs to develop muscle, it won't matter.

The greatest outcomes are obtained when food and exercise are combined, as opposed to when they are done individually. Utilize your exercise regimen to burn more calories, and your food to properly supply your body with the nutrients it needs to grow muscle. A pound of muscle weighs less than a pound of fat, I've heard numerous times throughout my life. A pound is a pound, even though this is untrue; a pound of muscle takes up less space on the body than a pound of fat. I would much rather have muscle than fat in my body, pound for pound. You would be well to keep in mind that dieting alone will not result in the development of muscle in your efforts.

You should also be aware that even though your weight may not be changing much while you gain muscle, you may be losing inches. You must keep this in mind at all times when trying to lose weight. You won't get accurate results if you just use the scales to gauge your progress. The issue is that a lot of individuals respond in this manner, becoming upset and giving up while they are truly moving forward. Don't let the scales win and make you a victim. Try on your tight jeans, look in the mirror, and take your waist measurement. Instead of focusing on the many pounds you lost this week, gauge your achievement by how you feel after ascending a flight of steps.

You may help your body burn off any excess calories you may have ingested throughout the day by including exercise in your eating plan. In other words, if you want to indulge in a minor "cheat" throughout the day, you may make up for it by burning a few more calories later on. Even while it shouldn't happen often, a single instance won't make or break your diet.

You should see the link between exercise and dieting as a match made in heaven. While it is possible to play baseball without a glove, doing so appears to function so much more effectively. For individuals who mix diet and exercise seriously, the outcomes for weight reduction may be amazing. Keep in mind that neither one works as well on its own and that neither one will function unless you are prepared to put in the necessary effort. To get the greatest outcomes, you must prioritize this in your life.

Chapter 13

DIETING WITHOUT SACRIFICE

So many people view dieting as some sort of cosmic punishment for not having the perfect body. They believe that enjoying food is somehow bad for them, which couldn't be further from the truth. If you want to be completely honest with yourself, when it comes to dieting, it isn't about giving up food or flavor; it's about discovering new foods and flavors. At least that is what it is for those who truly love food as well as adventure.

There are many spices out there that can make even the blandest of foods a little exciting. Fish and chicken are popular diet foods because they are lean meats. However, adding a little blackening seasoning is a great way to put a little punch in your meal that will make it taste great without packing on the calories of dressing marinades or soaking in butter before broiling. You do not have to stop there. Italian seasoning can also add a little flavor to your kitchen without adding the extra calories that you are working so hard to avoid.

All kinds of seasonings will work well in this instance. Many great seasonings for chicken also make great additions to chicken that will be included in salads for healthier lunches or salad wraps. Grains are good for you when you concentrate on whole grains. They are quite often the primary source of fiber in a diet and you need fiber almost as much as you need water. At any rate, simple things that spice up the same old lunch can have a huge impact on your enjoyment of food.

You can even enjoy the occasional treat when dieting as long as you do so sparingly. The key when dieting is to learn about proper portions and moderate indulgence. You can find all kinds of low-sugar or low-carb desserts on the market that you can enjoy sparingly. You can even find sugar-free or low-calorie candy in some cases though you should keep in mind that calories, particularly when it comes to candy you eat unconsciously add up quickly and you must pay close attention to those things you put into your mouth.

My point in all this though is that you do not have to sacrifice flavor to diet. You can live without butter; there are many substitutions on the market that are quite remarkable. But seasonings are a great way to add a lot of flavor for a tiny bit of effort on your part.

Desserts are also great and you can find many dips and sauces that can be made with fat-free or low-fat mayonnaise or sour cream to cut a few more calories during your dieting process.

These dips and sauces can often make a great substitution, when paired with vegetables, for those chips and dips we love so much and often miss when dieting. Cucumbers, green, red, and yellow peppers, broccoli, and carrot sticks all have a nice little crunch to them that when combined with a good low-fat dip can help cure the craving beast for greasy chips that often rears its head when dieting.

If you watch your calories carefully during meals you should be delighted to know that many little snack treats are prepackaged in 100-calorie packs for your enjoyment. This means that you can indulge on occasion in those treats that you love most without sacrificing all your dieting efforts in the process. These snack packs have become one of the best marketing ploys since the invention of diet colas. We all want the benefits of losing weight and will readily admit that if it were a simple process we'd all be thin. However, having something like these hundred-calorie snack packs to carry you through the worst of your cravings can mean the difference between dieting success and failure. They are a difference between the old way of dieting and the new way of dieting without sacrificing flavor.

Chapter 14

DIETING FOR FERTILITY

Obesity has many negative health consequences. Some are better known and documented than others. Recent studies have shown that yet another potential consequence of obesity is a difficulty when it comes to conceiving a baby. Fertility troubles are a growing problem in this country and around the world. One reason that is being hailed as a very viable culprit is obesity.

While most people look immediately to the female in the relationship for this particular problem the facts indicate that male obesity can also lead to a low sperm count, which can also hamper fertility efforts and progress.

Our bodies were designed for specific purposes. It is utterly amazing how well each part of the human body works to support the others. There are very few machines that can compete with the genius of the design of the human body. After thousands of years to study the human body there are still many mysteries hidden within. The truth comes down to this however, we put things into our bodies and abuse our bodies in ways that our bodies were simply not designed to take and yet we still manage to adapt and survive many of these things.

It's amazing when you think that the human body endures the many things it does without permanent and irrevocable damage. The good news for those attempting to conceive is that the human body also has the remarkable ability to heal itself. This means that those who find their efforts to conceive have been hampered by obesity have also seen positive changes by losing as little as five to ten percent of their ability to conceive.

If both partners are overweight then it might be a good idea to work together to shed those unwanted pounds and adopt a healthier, more active lifestyle. Being active when trying to conceive and throughout the pregnancy is a good idea for the female in the relationship at any rate as this can help in the process of labor and delivery.

If you are trying to conceive without success and have been doing so for more than a year it is probably in your best interest to seek the services of a fertility specialist to rule out other possible considerations. Though it is rarely a bad idea to adopt a healthier lifestyle you should also consult your doctor before beginning a strict diet or weight loss regimen to make sure there aren't other factors that may be causing your weight issues. This is particularly true if you have gained a good deal of weight in a rather short amount of time.

In addition to conception difficulty obesity can also lead to a greater risk of miscarriage once conception has occurred. Obesity also leads to a greater risk of conditions such as gestational diabetes during pregnancy, pre-eclampsia, and in some cases still birth and birth defects. It is no small hindrance to a healthy pregnancy and should be carefully considered before attempting to conceive.

Another consideration when it comes to obesity and fertility is that being overweight can also hamper the effects of fertility treatments. This means that the process is typically lengthier and will cost significantly more over time than if obesity were not a factor. When coupled with the risks to the baby this is something that should not be taken lightly when making plans for fertility treatments.

If your BMI is greater than 30 many fertility clinics simply will not offer their services. Some limit it to greater than 35 and others 40. If you feel that fertility treatments are the only course of action available to you and your BMI is greater than 30, the first suggestion you are likely to hear is the suggestion that you make serious weight loss efforts and lifestyle changes before proceeding. You may find that once you begin to shed pounds, fertility intervention is no longer necessary.

Chapter 15

HEALTHY DIETING TIPS

When it comes to dieting you will find all kinds of crazy and faddish diets on the market today. In addition to the many diets, there seems to be every kind of diet aid you can imagine. From shakes, the diet industry has evolved to include everything from candy bars and pudding to pills and patches. Each item claims that it can help you drop those unwanted pounds quickly and easily. Well, I can tell you for a fact there is very little easy for most of us about dropping a few pounds.

If you would like a few tips that should make your weight loss goals a little easier to achieve then perhaps the following tips will help you out.

Drink Plenty of Water

There isn't enough that can be said about the importance of drinking water to reach your fitness goals. Water hydrates the body first and foremost but water is also an important way of tricking your body into believing it is full. Other drinks do not work nearly as well as water in this endeavor and many drinks, even fruit juices, contain empty calories that you can ill afford when dieting.

Another great thing about drinking a lot of water while dieting is that it helps your skin retain its elasticity so you can avoid some of the 'loose skin' looks that often accompany massive weight loss. As a bonus drinking, plenty of water will make your skin look radiant and beautiful as well.

Set Goals

Having goals is one of the most important things you can do when working to lose weight. Try to make sure that your goals are aggressive but can be achieved. If you are frustrated early in the dieting process by unrealistic goals you are much more likely to give up. However, challenges are always going to inspire us to achieve greater things in life. If you can find a ‘weight loss partner to have a little friendly competition for the weight loss totals for a week or a month then you are going to be far more likely to accomplish your goals than if you keep them quietly to yourself.

Eat More

Did you read that twice? Yes, eat more healthy foods that are high in fiber. Eat more vegetables and fruits- fill up on these foods that are good for you and you will not be inclined to binge on calorie-laden junk food.

Move!

While this seems a little too simply stated for most, getting up and moving is one of, if not the absolute best way to burn calories. The simple truth is that you are not going to lose weight unless you use more calories than you consume. The more activities you enjoy that burn calorie, the more likely you are to shed those unwanted pounds and meet your weight loss goals.

Some great activities that burn calories include the following: gardening, golf, dancing, playing volleyball, walking, jumping rope, playing hopscotch with your little ones, and playing tennis. I mention these activities because you can trick yourself into believing that you aren't exercising while burning calories. Even cleaning the house requires movement and energy and if you dance around a little to some good music in the process you might burn a few extra calories.

Dieting, when successful, can help restore self-image and self-esteem in people who are otherwise beautiful inside and out. The steps above are not the only things that are involved in the dieting process but they can help you reach your weight loss goals, particularly when combined with a diet plan that you feel confident you can follow. Be sure that on those days when willpower is non-existent that you do not derail your diet efforts altogether by giving up. The most important thing you can do when dieting is to go back to dieting once you've strayed.

Chapter 16

FINDING THE BEAUTY WITHIN WHILE DIETING

There seems to be one universal truth when it comes to dieting. No one enjoys the process though we all eagerly await and anticipate the results. The problem is that far too many men and women around the world focus so much on dieting and perfecting their external beauty that they forget the beautiful people they are inside along the way. Our culture is becoming obsessive about the perfect body and the perfect body image.

If there was one message that should make it out to everyone dieing it is this: dieting should be more about health than beauty. You should not need to conform to some preconceived notion of what is or should be beautiful. If we create a world where everyone looks alike it would be rather boring in the end.

You need to focus on being happy with who you are to achieve the greatest dieting success you will have ever dared dream of. Many of us eat out of emotional need or a simple need for comfort when we are depressed, hurting, uncertain, or simply in unfamiliar territory. No solution will work for everyone when it comes to making peace with who you are and this by no means indicates that you should no longer seek to be the healthiest you there is. It simply means that your focus should be more on coming to terms with who you are as a person than on creating a new person or image behind which you can hide.

Dieting for the most part is an opportunity for many men and women to become someone else. Whether that someone is the person you used to be or some person you think you want to be, you are quite unlikely to find happiness at any weight until you accept yourself for the person you are inside. This is often a difficult process but one that is well worth the effort. Once you've accepted the person inside you can address the specific needs that often lead to excess weight, to begin with. Depression is a common factor in weight gain as well as an inability to lose weight. By finding contentment depression will no longer be a controlling factor in your life. For many, this is the freedom they need from their weight problems while others will find there are still hurdles remaining.

The important thing is that you stop allowing the person you are to be defined by what the scales say about you. Once you've reached a point in your life where you are happy with your appearance and feel that your fitness level is in hand you should discuss things with your doctor and see what he or she has to say. We do not need a nation of size 5 women. We need a nation of women who are self-aware and self-confident and not afraid to be who they are on the inside regardless of how they look on the outside.

Finding the beauty within is often the most important aspect of dieting that there can be. Take the time while dieting to get to know the person you are and introduce that person to the person you want to be. In time the two will work out a healthy compromise and you will find that image isn't everything no matter what the glossy magazines try to tell you.

www.ingramcontent.com/pod-product-compliance
Lightning Source LLC
LaVergne TN
LVHW012113160826
845678LV00014B/3077

* 9 7 9 8 3 6 1 6 9 4 6 0 0 *